Childhood Obesity Prevention And Treatment

Eating Healthy Can Be Fun!

By Natalie Johnson

Table of Contents

Introduction

I want to thank you and congratulate you for downloading the book, Childhood Obesity Prevention and Treatment: Eating Healthy Can Be Fun!

Obesity is not only a problem that attacks adults; children are also susceptible to this health condition. In fact, children may even be at a higher risk of getting obese. A parent's overwhelming love for their child and feeding them with more than enough can be the start of such problem.

This problem though, even if it's genetically caused, is not impossible to solve. What you just need to know are the steps on how to accomplish it.

This book will tackle the problem of obesity in children. The first chapter will focus on its causes and health risks that the condition poses on the child. The succeeding chapters will then focus on the time tested trifecta in combating obesity – family support and encouragement, being mindful of what and how you eat, and physical activities. All of these are tailored so that it can fit the needs of a child.

Enjoy the book, and we hope that you may also adapt these practices in your life to stay healthy just like your   child.

Chapter 1
Is your child cute or obese? :
Know when to draw the line

We all know that children are cute and irresistible. They become more so when they look healthy. This is why many parents strive to give the food that their child wants. However, an excess of something is not good. This can even lead to childhood obesity – and this situation is not cute.

This chapter will present about childhood obesity, along with other relevant information that will help parents understand more about it.

What is childhood obesity?

This condition is like obesity in adulthood – just experienced by children. It is said that a child is obese if they have excess body fat that can bring negative consequences to their well-being.

How will you know if your child is obese?

Computing for the Body Mass Index (BMI) is a reliable method used to determine if an individual (adult or child alike) is obese. However, there are some deviations from how the BMI for children is computed as compared to adults.

BMI for adults are computed based on a formula that will be applied on the person's weight and height. For children, however, the BMI is based on a growth chart. Because a child's physical growth is rapid and it follows a pattern, it is easy to detect if their weight is under the normal range. If the child's weight falls on the 85th percentile, they are then considered as overweight. If the child's weight reaches the 95th percentile, that's the only time that they're called obese.

It is best to consult a physician to ascertain if your child is obese or not, and not consult based on your child's weight alone. This is because not all children whose weight is under the "overweight" or "obese" category need to lose weight. The physician also needs to determine if the child's weight is caused by fat in the body (as there are children who weigh as such because their body has lean tissue or heavier bones).

Health risks of childhood obesity

Being obese alone is a health risk itself. However, the child is also exposed to other health risks that obesity brings along with it.

The following is a list of other health conditions that an obese child may develop and experience:

- Emotional and/or psychological problem – obese children are observed to have low self-esteem. Their difference in body weight can cause them to be envious of other children who are able to do things (such as being active) that they cannot do because their body prevents them from engaging in it. This can lead to few friends and less social interaction – things that your child needs to develop their interpersonal skills. They may also experience teasing and bullying.

• High blood pressure and heart disease – fats are caused by cholesterol, which can block arteries if the body has an excess of it.

• Increased risk for diabetes – another cause of fat accumulation is the excessive consumption of foods that are rich in sugar (such as candies or chocolates). If your child's body accumulates too much sugar in the blood, this can cause diabetes. And this condition may be far worse than obesity; it can be inherited, and it will not go away even if the child gets rid of his/her obesity.

• Sleep problems – too much food intake can cause the pancreas to work overtime, leading to difficulty initiating sleep (since the body's processes are slower at night).

- Joint and bone problems – the bones and joints of your child may not withstand the weight that it has to carry. This can lead to difficulties in moving from one place to another, even if it's only for a short distance.

What causes childhood obesity?

The following situations can cause a child to become obese:

- Too much food intake – although eating is necessary to provide your child's body with the energy that it will need to function properly, eating too much will bring unnecessary fat to their body, hence leading to more weight.

- Lack of exercise or physical activity – this, along with too much food intake, is the deadly combination for childhood obesity. As long as the body is able to use up most of the energy that it has stored, fat will never accumulate (since physical activity will "burn" the fat).

- Easy access to high-calorie junk food and fast food – these foods serve as "catalysts" of obesity, especially if your child is able to consume them regularly. Since fast food stores grow at a fast pace and junk foods are all around the market, children have easier access to them. They are even used by parents as "reward" just for their children to behave accordingly.

- Genes – some children may accumulate more weight than others due to their genetic make-up. It may be caused by different conditions which include being overweight/obese in its symptoms.

Busting myths about childhood obesity

There are certain "incorrect beliefs" that parents hold when it comes to their child's weight. This section will "bust" some myths and present the facts about them.

- Most parents believe that if the cause of their child's obesity is their genes, they can't do something to counter their inevitable weight gain. Although it is true that they might gain weight faster even when there is moderate food intake, it is still possible for them to maintain a healthy weight. They just need to exercise and eat right.

- Most parents do not believe that their child is obese. According to them, their child only has baby fat – which they will eventually outgrow. However, this is not true in all cases. Not giving attention to your child's weight, thinking that it will eventually normalize, can lead to a significant increase to the child's tendency to become obese until adulthood.

- If parents have determined that their child is obese, most of them take drastic measures – specifically, putting them on a diet. Although it is true that monitoring your child's food intake can affect their weight, this action should not always be used unless it is advised by your doctor. Unless necessary, the goal of treatment is not to lose weight; rather, it is for them to stop or slow down the weight gain. By doing so, the weight that is considered "overweight" before might be considered as normal after some years (since there will be a balance on the height and weight of your child).

Now that the basics have been covered, this book will now proceed on actions that can be taken to treat or even prevent your child from being obese.

Chapter 2
Family involvement:
How it can help manage your child's weight

Even if it's your child alone that's experiencing the problems associated with obesity, it doesn't mean that the family will never do something about it. In order to manage your child's weight faster, what they need is support and involvement from the family.

This chapter will highlight the steps that your family can adapt in order to help your child in managing their weight problem.

Be an example

As a parent, you are the first source of your child when it comes to almost everything – including their diet. Hence, if you want to influence them to adapt a healthy habit, you need to be their "model". Not only will you help your child to manage their weight, you also become conscious of yours and help you to also stay healthy.

You can accomplish this by adapting the following habits:

- Invite your child to consume healthy food while you're eating it yourself – if you want them to adapt the habit of eating healthy food, they need to see you do it first. By doing so, they will get the idea that you value eating healthy food and you want them to adapt that same healthy habit.

- Cook healthy recipes in front of them and employ their help while you're cooking – children will become more interested in eating the food if they became part of the process in preparing it. The time while cooking can also be a short session about the food you're cooking and the health benefits they can get by consuming it.

- Refrain from "sedentary" relaxation – even your free time can be used to teach your child something about health. One good behavior that you should adapt is to avoid getting in front of the television or computer for a considerable amount of time. It would be better if you can spend your free time together while staying active. If you're not into sports, you can accomplish household tasks such as gardening (which also requires physical activity). This will help your child to engage in a productive task while making sure that his body is active (and is burning unwanted fats).

- Make small changes when adapting new healthy habits – introducing a new healthy habit is not easy, especially if the habit requires effort. Hence, if you want to reach this goal, you can start with taking "small steps" towards it. Suggest with a small activity that your family members will most likely participate in (such as taking a walk outside after dinner) before inviting them to engage in an activity that requires more physical effort (such as participating in a marathon). The chance that your family members will participate in the larger favor increases by asking them to participate with a small one first.

Be informed about your child's life

You can be further involved with your child if you're updated with whatever is happening to him/her.

Here are some of the habits that you can adapt in order for you to be updated with your child's life.

- Listen to your child and speak with his/her teachers – obese children are prone to being bullied. In order to save your child from experiencing such, you need to make your child feel that you're there for him/her. Listening to any of his/her concerns will foster trust between the two of you, which in the long run will be helpful in developing their self-esteem and making them more motivated to deal with their weight issues. Speaking with their teachers can also help you in getting updated if ever your child is "clamming up" (not willing to share information with you).

- Always make sure that you have time for them – although it may be hard to find time for chit-chat, you need to allot enough time so you can attend to them. Treat is as a very important meeting or appointment that you can never afford to miss. This also aims to boost their self-esteem and start making positive changes.

The amount of support and involvement that the family provides to the obese child is important if they want the child to solve their "heavy" problem. After all, any burden is light if more people will carry it.

Chapter 3

Intelligent food choices for weight management

Food is the primary contributor of both nutrition and fat in an individual's body. Hence, the kind of food that your child eats determines how their weight will turn out (if they will lose, maintain, or gain weight).

This chapter will focus on what you need to know about food – specifically, what you eat and its amount – that will be beneficial for weight management.

Healthier food choices and habits

Reaching your ideal weight is not a walk in the park, primarily because you need to implement major changes on the diet that you've gotten used to. Although it is common knowledge that you need to eat healthy if you want to stay healthy, most people do not know where to start.

The following tips will guide your child to the right path towards healthier weight:

- Eat breakfast! – make it a priority to never let your child skip breakfast, and make sure that they're eating the right kinds of food such as whole grain cereals, low fat milk, or oatmeal. This helps prevent your child's body from cravings for high-sugar foods. Although the latter can give them energy, high-sugar foods are easily exhausted by the body; hence, they will need an additional meal just to get through the morning.

- Foods with rainbow colors are the best – nutritionists believe that foods whose colors can be found in the rainbow will do wonders for your health (and also weight). Hence, obese children should be encouraged to eat a wide variety of fruits and vegetables if they want to stay healthy and reach their ideal weight. Since children can easily memorize the colors of the rainbow, they can easily determine if the food that they will eat can promote their health.

- Know about healthy fats – most people simply know that fat should be limited to their diet. However, there is such thing as "healthy fat", and these are necessary in our bodies. Fats such as monounsaturated and polyunsaturated fats are essential acids that our body needs for good health. Fish and nuts are good sources of these healthy fats.

- Introduce a meal time schedule – most obese children do not have control as to what time they will eat; as long as they're hungry, they will eat something even if it's just a few minutes before lunch or dinner. By introducing a specific time when they should eat, they are more likely to eat what you give to them and not be picky about food (as children will always prefer candy over fruits or vegetables). This also reduces the number of meals that they will have throughout the day.

- Dine out less – consumerism sometimes influence parents to take the "easy route"; meaning, dine out rather than prepare meals at home. After all, not everyone has the time. However, dining out (especially in fast food establishments) can make you miss on nutrients that are present on their counterparts. Preparing food at home is not only a good time to strengthen your relationships; it will also help you save money and be in control of the nutrients that you want your child to intake.

Guidelines for snacks and sweets

Children are naturally attracted to sweets. However, the consumption of these foods can cause childhood obesity. Therefore, as their parent, it is your duty to set the guidelines for the consumption of these treats.

The following rules can be set when it comes to the consumption of sweets and snacks:

- Snacks should never be a meal – if you're offering snacks, make sure that its serving is not equal to a usual meal. Snacks are meant to give you a short boost of energy that you can use if ever the energy you've gained during your previous meal was running out. Hence, their calorie content should not be as large as a meal. Make sure that the snack you'll be giving will not exceed 150 calories (which is enough for your body to stay satiated for 1 to 2 hours, depending on the activity). By doing so, your child can avoid calorie surplus and weight gain.

- Juice and sodas should be limited – sodas are packed with "empty sugars" that doesn't have a contribution to your child's health. Juices, especially powdered ones, are also the same. Instead of giving these to your children, you can offer healthier alternatives such as fruit juices or fruit smoothies.

- Fruit-based snacks should be the focus of your child's diet – although they are not as sweet as sugar-based snacks such as chocolates or candies, fruit-based snacks are healthier alternatives as compared to the former. They can be used to replace candies for dessert; and if prepared creatively, they can be attractive for your child to consume as a snack as well. Frozen bananas, strawberries and yogurt, and sliced apples with peanut butter are examples of these sweet but healthy alternatives.

- "No sweet" rules should never be implemented – you can never deprive your child to consume what they like. This is because if you do, they will overindulge on the sweets if ever they got the chance. Aside from the fruit-based alternatives, you can still offer candies. However, you need to limit your child's intake so that it stays within the healthy range of calories that they are consuming. In time, they will get used to fruit-based desserts and snacks and consume minimum amounts of sugar-based foods.

Serving sizes matter

Aside from "lower sweets, higher fruit and vegetable" consumption, you also need to monitor the serving portion of your child when eating.

The following tips regarding portion sizes can also be applied to your child:

- Check the food label – important information such as serving size and the nutrients that the food contains are all found on the food label. Check for its calorie content and the recommended portion size.

- Food in large packages should be divided into smaller containers – this is done to prevent overconsumption. Your child will fail to realize that they consumed a lot already if it is not transferred to a smaller container (since the content doesn't seem to be depleting if it remains in the large packaging).

- Meals should be served in individual plates – if you want to minimize the amount of food that your child will consume, make sure to serve the food directly in their plate rather than prepare serving dishes. This will minimize their tendency to reach for another helping.

- Use smaller plates – preparing your child's meals in a smaller plate will create the impression that they have eaten enough (since even a small amount of food can look overwhelming if served in a small plate).

- If ever you'll be eating out, reduce your orders – if you're used to ordering full servings for a dish, make sure that you order smaller portions than what you've gotten used to. Or better yet, you can share with your child and order one serving instead of two. This will significantly reduce the amount of food and calories that they will consume.

Chapter 4

Program of activities for your child's weight management

Another important factor that can help your obese child to get back on the normal weight range, they need to get their body to work.

This chapter will focus on the activities that your child can participate in for them to manage their weight problem.

Exercise idea for your child

Exercise is not only limited to hitting the gym and lifting weights. For children, exercise means getting enough physical activity so that their fats are burned and the energy they've gained from food expended.

Here are some that you can do so that your child can get the exercise that they need:

- Get him outside – the first major step that parents should take is to entice their children into going outside. This is because many children are content with staying at home and playing with their gadgets rather than experience playing in real life. Not only can it help burn fat, it can also improve some of their skills (such as running, catching, etc.) and improve their stamina.

- Add a little physical activity into your indoor games – if you have difficulty convincing your child to play outside, or if you live in a neighborhood that can be dangerous for them (your house is located beside the street), you can play active games inside the house. Games such as hide and seek or crawling tag (to reduce the risk of mess all over the house) can give the same effect as playing outside.

- If your child is not born for too much physical activity (he/she has asthma or other conditions), you can focus on assigning household chores that are appropriate for their age. Surprisingly, there are a number of chores that can burn a significant amount of calories – this includes vacuuming, sweeping, mopping, and mowing the lawn.

- Talk to your child about an after-school sport or activity that they want to engage in – if you have sufficient money, you can choose to enroll them in a sports class or any physically inclined activity that they can attend to after school. Ask them about the activity that they want to participate in, and tell them that participating in it can serve as their stress reliever after studying the whole day. They also get to explore the fields where they can gain proficiency and significantly boost their self-esteem.

Replacing "screen time" with "exercise time"

TV became the nanny of the modern parent. Since their child's attention is shifted to the screen, parents are able to focus on their work without interference. However, this created a problem – that is, children become more interested in watching shows rather than going outside. This inactivity, coupled with incorrect diet, is what causes obesity in children.

Therefore, it is important for parents to reduce the time that their child spends in front of the screen and replace it with exercise.

Here are some of the steps that they can follow to achieve this goal:

- Reduce the number of hours watching – set a maximum of 2 hours per day limit that your child is allowed to watch the TV. This is because recent researches show that those who spend too much time in front of the TV have a larger tendency to become obese.

- Never eat in front of the TV – since TV catches your child's attention, they will not be able to monitor the amount of food that they've already consumed, making them more prone to eat more than what they're supposed to. This routine also ruins the time that's supposed to be allotted for the family.

- Never use TV time as a reward or punishment – reducing or increasing time in watching TV just to punish or reinforce behavior is not helpful. In fact, you're only reinforcing that TV is important, and they can get time to watch TV if they follow what you say. Instead of TV time, you can promise something else. This can be an outdoor activity that you will both enjoy, or grant one wish that can be beneficial to your child.

Once you got to reduce the amount of time that your child spends in front of the TV, that's the time when you can introduce the exercise ideas mentioned earlier. These activities will then replace the "screen time" that your child has been spending before.

Conclusion

Fighting obesity is not a hard task to accomplish. As long as you can start on the right path and be consistent with your effort to help your child achieve their ideal weight, it is not impossible.

Since children do not fully understand what obesity can bring them if they don't do something about it, it is your job as their parent to guide them and teach habits that will help them in achieving a healthier body.

We hope that this book can lighten the burden that you've been experiencing with your child. We also hope that you can apply it in yourself and prevent obesity.

Finally, if you enjoyed this book, please take the time to share your thoughts and post a review on Amazon. It'd be greatly appreciated!

www.ingramcontent.com/pod-product-compliance
Lightning Source LLC
Chambersburg PA
CBHW061933280526
45787CB00004B/1594